Stop Gout

An Essential Guide to Reducing Inflammation

Contains: Gout Prevention – Gout Treatment – Gout Diet

Gout Relief – Anti Inflammation 7 Day Meal Plan – Anti Inflammatory Recipes & more

JT Thorpe

Gout 6

Facts about Gout 8

Prevalence of Gout 15

Death from Gout 17

Causes of Gout 21

Triggers of Gout 22

Treatment of Gout 29

Medications for an Acute Attack of Gout 33

Medications for decreasing Uric Acid Levels 37

Self-Care for Gout 42

Dietary Goals 43

Physical Activity to reduce Gouty Attacks 46

Complications of Gout 47

Alternative Medications for Gouty Arthritis 51

Prevention of Gout 54

Exercises for Gout 59

Aerobic Exercise 62

Natural Supplements for Gout 65

Dealing with a Loved One with Gout 72

Gout Resources 74

Misinformation about Gout 77

Side Effects from Gout Drugs 84

Case Study on Gout 92

Anti Inflammation 101

So what is inflammation? 103

Signs of Inflammation: 105

Diet 109

Fat 110

Protein 112

Carbohydrates 113

Herbs and Spices 115

Beverages 117

Putting It All Together 120

Foods to Limit and/or Avoid in Your Diet 121

So What to Eat Instead? 124

Nuts and Seeds 125

Colorful fruits and vegetables 126

Olive Oil 126

Beans 127

Recipes 133

Spinach and Mushroom Frittata 133

Coconut Quinoa Porridge with Ginger and Dates 135

Shrimp and vegetable soup 136

Drunken Mussels 137

Pecan Rosemary Baked Tilapia 139

Fennel, Apple and Celery Salad 141

Tips for adjusting to a new diet 142

The Best (and Healthiest) Ways to Indulge 144

Mexican Hot Chocolate 144

Grilled fruit 145

Banana "Ice Cream" with Cinnamon and Walnuts 145

Baked Ricotta with Berries 146

The Lifestyle Changes That Will Reduce Inflammation
147

Lose Weight 149

Reduce Blood Sugar 153

Avoid Repetitive Motions 159

Reduce Stress 161

Preventing Stress 164

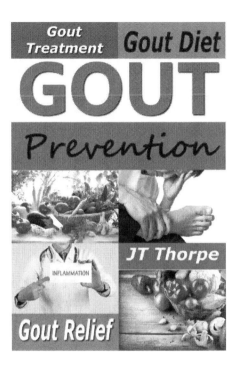

Gout Prevention

Gout Treatment

Gout Diet

Gout Relief

©All Rights Reserved

JT Thorpe

Gout

Gout is a type of joint disease that is linked to the buildup of uric acid crystals in the fluids and tissues inside the body. It can be caused by the kidneys not being able to excrete uric acid from the body or from an overproduction of uric acid in the body. It is generally related to a poor diet, alcohol consumption, and the taking of certain medications, yet there are hereditary forms of the disease as well. There are about 3 million Americans who currently live with gout or gouty arthritis.

When a person suffers from acute gout, they may have a specific joint that becomes hot, swollen and red. The joint pain Is usually unilateral, meaning it doesn't affect the same joint on both sides of the body.

Most people with acute gout suffer from excruciating pain in the affected joint that can be easily managed by taking some type of NSAID drug (nonsteroidal anti-inflammatory drug) such as ibuprofen (marketed as Motrin or Advil) or naproxen sodium (marketed as Naprosyn or Aleve). Changes in diet and preventative medications can prevent an acute flare-up of gout but when a flare-up occurs, medications are generally necessary.

If acute gout is left untreated and the individual has repetitive instances of gout, this can cause a degenerative type of gout in the joints, which is also referred to as chronic gout or gouty arthritis. The goal of treatment in those suffering from gouty arthritis is to treat the pain of flare-ups and to keep the uric acid levels down as much as possible.

Facts about Gout

- Gout has been around for millennia and has been recorded ancient medical texts.

- Gouty arthritis is the most common type of arthritis due to inflammation in men.

- Gout is defined as having elevated uric acid levels that cause acute flare-ups of gouty arthritis interspersed with periods of remission, although some men can suffer from chronic gouty arthritis that does not have a period of remission associated with it.

- The main cause of gout is an elevated uric acid level.

- High levels of uric acid cause monosodium urate crystals to become deposited in the tissues.

- Gouty arthritis from elevated uric acid levels is secondary to high levels of uric acid in the joint tissues themselves.

- Uric acid is the end product of the metabolism of purines in the diet.

- Purines can be found in several types of foods, such as red meat. Purines can also be found as a part of normal human tissues.

- The presence of high uric acid levels is called "hyperuricemia". It can be caused by a lack of balance between the excretion of uric acid by the kidneys and the making too much uric acid in the tissues.

- While all cases of gout are caused by elevated uric acid in the system, not all cases of elevated uric acid will lead to gout.

- If a person simply has high uric acid levels, treatment is unnecessary unless symptoms are present.

- Common reasons why a person might get gout include being obese or overweight, having high blood pressure, drinking beer and other alcoholic beverages (except wine), diets high in red meat or seafood, and poor kidneys.

- Gout can be managed in part by losing weight.

There are typically several stages in gout. These include the following:

- The deposition of uric acid in the tissues in the absence of any type of symptoms.

• Acute flare-ups occurring when the uric acid in the joints cause inflammation in the joint tissues. The most common flare-up will occur in the lower extremity joints. During an acute flare-up of the disease, the joints are painful, red, swollen and warm. This can last for several days up to several weeks.

• The most common location of an acute flare-up is the first metatarsophalangeal joint, which is the joint that connects the big toe to the rest of the foot. About half of all cases of gouty arthritis occur in this joint. Approximately 80 percent of patients with gout will have arthritis in this joint.

• Half of the patients with the clinical findings of gout will have a normal uric acid level, which makes the diagnosis difficult. It can be especially difficult to diagnose in the elderly patient, who usually will present atypically with more than a single affected joint.

• In between flare-ups, the person may have elevated uric acid levels without any of the typical symptoms of gout.

• As the disease progresses, there are fewer periods in which the patient is asymptomatic.

• If the individual is suffering from chronic gout, there is a constant arthritis of the joints, in which the pain does not let up.

- In very severe cases, the individual can develop tophi, which are clumps of uric acid crystals in the soft tissue around the joints. Tophi are most common in the finger joints, ears, and elbows. These tend to be areas of the body that are cooler than other areas of the body.

- People with gout have a higher than normal risk of having kidney stones.

- The best way to diagnose gout is to take a sampling of the effusion around the joint and looking under the microscope for uric acid crystals within the joint fluid. The presence of tophi can also help make the diagnosis of gout.

- The basic treatment for gout includes treating the pain associated with gouty arthritis and preventing more attacks of gouty arthritis by keeping the uric acid levels as low as possible.

- Common treatments for acute flare-ups include NSAID therapy, colchicine, and corticosteroids. One can also prevent flare-ups by reducing the weight, staying away from alcohol, and taking drugs that lower the risk of hyperuricemia (elevated uric acid levels).

Prevalence of Gout

The term "prevalence" means the number patient living with gout, regardless of whether the gouty symptoms are new or not. About 3.9 percent of Americans are currently living with gout. In men, the prevalence is higher at 5.9 percent. If the patient is a woman, the prevalence of gout is much less at only 2 percent. The prevalence of gout has increased in the last twenty years by 1.2 percent.

Incidence of Gout

The incidence of gout is defined as the number of new cases of gout each year. According to statistics compiled by the CDC, black men have twice the incidence of gout when compared to Caucasians. The incidence of gout among black men is 10.9 percent with an incidence of gout in white men being only 5.8 percent.

According to statistics compiled by the Rochester Epidemiology Project, there has been an increase in the incidence of gout between the latter half of the 1970s and the latter half of the 1990s. There was an incidence of gout of 45 per 100,000 individuals in the late 1970s. This number increased to 63.3 per 100,000 individuals in the late 1990s. If the individual had primary gouty arthritis (arthritis not due to diuretic use), this incidence increased from 20.2 per 100,000 people to 45.9 per 100,000 people during the twenty years between the 1970s and the 1990s.

Death from Gout

Researchers looking at information from the Health Professionals Follow-Up Study discovered that men suffering from gout have a greater than average risk of dying from any cause. The main cause of death in men who have gout is cardiovascular disease. The chances of dying from any cause among people who have gout has a ratio of 1.38:1. It should be noted that these people are not usually dying from gout. It just means that these people have related risk factors (such as obesity and heart disease) that puts them at a greater risk of dying.

Symptoms of Gout As mentioned, just the presence of elevated uric acid levels doesn't mean you have gout and there are few symptoms. When gout has advanced to become symptomatic, the first symptom is usually the development of exquisite pain and swelling of the metatarsophalangeal joint of the great toe. It can come out of the blue or can follow an acute injury or an illness, such as a viral or bacterial infection. While gouty arthritis usually affects the metatarsophalangeal joint of the great toe, it can also present itself as pain and inflammation of the knee joint or an ankle joint. Attacks of gouty arthritis can affect the same joint the second time around or can skip to another joint in the body. If left untreated, the acute attack of gouty arthritis turns into a chronic case of gouty arthritis, which is more difficult to treat.

Usually only one joint is affected at any given time unless the disease is untreated and is really out of control. The time of onset to the time of resolution of symptoms is about 7 to 10 days. The pain goes from being excruciating to a dull, constant pain in the joint.

Tophi come from gout that has been allowed to be unchecked for many years. Tophi are deposits of uric acid that generally cluster around a joint. Tophi can disfigure the joint so that it is difficult to work with the affected area. Tophi may be debilitating but they are generally not painful.

Another complication of severe gout is the presence of kidney stones. Kidney stones occur when the uric acid is excreted in large amounts by the kidneys. If the urine is really concentrated, the uric acid precipitates out into a crystal that grows to become a painful renal stone.

While things like an elevated blood pressure, obesity, chronic renal disease, heart disease, and diabetes are not directly related to having gout, these symptoms and diseases are often seen together along with elevated uric acid levels. The typical gout patient is a male who is obese and who lives a sedentary lifestyle. His intake is likely to be high in red meat.

Causes of Gout

While the symptoms of gout appear to happen overnight, the ongoing process leading up to a painful attack of gouty arthritis comes on over a process of many months or years. The most basic cause of gout is an elevation of uric acid in the body (hyperuricemia). This is brought on by eating a diet high in purines (red meat is an example) or by failing to excrete uric acid to an adequate degree by the kidneys.

Uric acid is a breakdown product of purines. Purines are made by cells of the body and are taken in as part of the diet. Under normal conditions, the uric acid breakdown product is sent from the cells of the body to the kidneys, where it is excreted. The sufferer of gout tends to make more purines or eat more purines in the diet or fails to excrete it due to kidney disease.

The main causes of gout include the following:

- Eating high purine-containing foods

- Being obese

- Drinking too much alcohol, particularly beer

- Living a sedentary lifestyle

Triggers of Gout

Hyperuricemia alone does not trigger gout. There often is another trigger in the individual's life that brings on the onset of a painful arthritic joint. There are medical triggers for gout. These include the following:

- Taking diuretic medications that concentrate the uric acid in the blood. Diuretics are used to treat high blood pressure, heart failure, or swelling of the legs.

- Infections occurring in the body, not necessarily in the joints of the body.

- The onset of a severe illness anywhere in the body.

- Injury to a specific joint that responds by precipitating uric acid crystals into the joint space.

- Being on chemotherapy drugs.

- Starting a medication that is supposed to reduce the uric acid in the blood.

- Taking cyclosporine for various reasons.

Some of the lifestyle factors that trigger gout include the following:

- Consumption of sugary beverages, such as sodas

- Dehydration through not taking in fluids or losing fluids through diarrhea or diuretics

- Taking on a crash diet or fasting

- Eating high purine foods, such as shellfish and red meats

- Drinking excessive amounts of alcohol, particularly beer

It is important to remember that these triggers lead to hyperuricemia, which may or may not result in gouty arthritis. Not all cases of hyperuricemia will be symptomatic and will lead to joint pain. This is why the absolute value of the uric acid is not a good diagnostic test for gouty arthritis as the elevation in uric acid may not be the cause of a given case of arthritis and gouty arthritis may be present with normal uric acid levels.

Risk Factors for Gout

As mentioned, about 3 million or more people in the US suffer from gout. Those at the highest risk of developing gout include the following:

- Men at any age, although the disease increases with age.

- Women who have already gone through menopause.

- People of any age with kidney disease.

- People who are obese.

- People who have high blood pressure.

- People with elevated cholesterol and triglyceride levels.

- People with diabetes.

- Having a family history of gout.

- Advancing age (gout is extremely rare in children but increases as one gets older).

The Diagnosis of Gout

If a uric acid level alone does not diagnose gout, there needs to be other ways of identifying a hot, red joint as being gouty arthritis. The doctor will ask you about your medical history and about your diet. Family history of gout may be asked about.

The doctor will check a uric acid level as part of the diagnosis and will examine the joint involved in an attempt to narrow down the diagnosis. The doctor will ask the following questions:

• What other symptoms are you experiencing?

• What medications are you currently taking?

• Are you taking a diuretic medication?

• What does the joint pain feel like?

• What is your diet like?

- How quickly did the symptoms come on?

- Does gout run in your family?

- Which joint or joints are affected?

The answers you give to these questions will help the doctor decide whether or not to pursue a more aggressive approach to diagnosing the type of arthritis you have.

The doctor may do exclusionary testing to make sure the arthritis is not from another cause. This may involve assessing the joint for infection by doing a CBC and perhaps a joint fluid culture or blood culture. X-rays may be taken to rule out other causes of arthritis. The serum uric acid level will be drawn even though it only partially helps make the diagnosis.

A CT scan or MRI scan of the joint may need to be performed to rule out other causes of arthritis. Ultrasounds of the joint may be helpful. The doctor may eventually take sample of the fluid around the joint. This fluid will be evaluated under the microscope for the presence of bacteria (in a bacterial arthritic condition) or for crystals of uric acid, which stand out under microscopic examination.

Uric acid crystals have a characteristic appearance that differentiate it from other crystal-related arthritis conditions, such as pseudo-gout. The presence of the classic crystals under a microscopic evaluation will clinch the diagnosis or gouty arthritis.

Treatment of Gout

Once gout takes hold and causes gouty arthritis, there are things that can be done to alleviate the pain and decrease the amount of inflammation in the affected joint. There is a two-way approach to the treatment of gouty arthritis that includes both the taking of medications to block inflammation and lifestyle changes to keep the uric acid levels low.

The treatment of an acute attack of gouty arthritis involves doing the following:

•   Take an NSAID medication. NSAIDs are nonsteroidal anti-inflammatory medications. They include ibuprofen and naproxen sodium, both of which are over the counter medications. Many doctors prescribe indomethacin, which is marketed as Indocin as this is a particularly strong NSAID medication that requires a prescription.   Acetaminophen (marketed as Tylenol) is not generally used as it only treats pain and does not affect inflammation.

•   Apply ice and Elevate the affected Joint. This is done so that the inflammation can settle down and the pain can be lessened. Whenever the affected joint is kept above the level of the heart, it throbs less and the pain is improved.

• Drink Plenty of fluids. Fluids can help flush the kidneys so you don't get kidney stones from a buildup of uric acid in the kidneys. Avoid sodas containing sugar and alcohol as these can make the arthritis worse.

• See your doctor. Because over the counter medications do not work as well as prescription medications for gouty arthritis, you may wish to see the doctor for prescription medications that can better alleviate the pain. Medications to reduce uric acid levels can also be given.

• Try to relax. Stress and anxiety can make gout symptoms worse so the more you relax, the less will be your perception of pain.

• Ask for help. You will need to have help with activities of daily living while you are laid up with gout. Ask friends and loved ones to do your chores for you so that you can take the time and heal from your condition.

Remember that, even though this is an extremely intense pain and you may feel as though it's the worst pain you have ever had, the attacks tend to peak at about 5-7 days and resolve themselves after about ten days. The first day and a half may be rough but this is usually the wore that it gets. As soon as you have an attack, see your doctor so as to resolve the symptoms as soon as possible so you can get back on your feet within about 10 days.

Medications for an Acute Attack of Gout

There are medications you can take to treat a gouty attack as soon as it has it has begun. Some are over the counter, while others can only be gotten by a prescription:

• NSAIDs. These are the nonsteroidal anti-inflammatory medications talked about above. They include ibuprofen (Advil, Aleve) and naproxen sodium (Naprosyn, Aleve). As mentioned, many doctors will prescribe prescription strength NSAID medications for you if you see the doctor. NSAIDs act to decrease inflammation and are best taken as soon as you know you are having an attack of gouty arthritis.

• Corticosteroids. This includes oral medications, such as prednisone, or injectable medications that are injected directly into the joint affected by gout. They act to decrease inflammation and can cut down on the swelling. They can be given intravenously if the gouty attack is very severe and doesn't seem to be getting any better with oral medications. If you have a gouty arthritis attack that affects more than one joint, which would make injecting each joint impractical.

• ACTH. ACTH is produced by the anterior pituitary gland and normally raises the corticosteroid levels in the body by acting on the adrenal gland. Your doctor can inject ACTH in order to cause the adrenal glands to put out more corticosteroids so that you don't need to take an injection of artificial corticosteroids. The body will naturally make its own corticosteroids that will decrease the inflammation of the affected joint. ACTH, just like injectable corticosteroids, will begin relieving your pain within about a day following the injection.

• Colchicine. Colchicine has been used for millennia in the treatment of gouty arthritis. It is a plant-derived medication that is used exclusively for the treatment of an acute attack of gouty arthritis. Be aware of side effects of this drug, which include abdominal pains, nausea, vomiting, and diarrhea. Some people can have more serious side effects from this drug so it should be used with caution and only under a doctor's supervision. Like other medications for gouty arthritis, it is best when it is used as soon as possible after you know you are suffering from an attack.

Medications for decreasing Uric Acid Levels

These medications are not very effective when you already have an acute attack of gouty arthritis and can, in fact, make the symptoms of gout worse during an attack. They are instead taken chronically once you know you have high uric acid levels. Because they can precipitate an attack of gouty arthritis, your doctor will often prescribe this class of medications after your attack is over with. They are mainly for decreasing uric acid levels in susceptible individuals.

Often, the doctor will prescribe a minimal dose of an NSAID medication or colchicine along with one of these medications to be used for several weeks and up to a year after your first attack to keep other attacks from occurring in the future.

These are the most common drugs used to decrease uric acid levels:

• Febuxostat. This is an anti-gout medication used to decrease uric acid levels in those people who do not tolerate allopurinol (described below) or who have some type of kidney disease. It works by decreasing the amount of uric acid produced by the body. Many doctors will start a low dose of the medication in the beginning to avoid side effects and will increase the amount of drug given if the uric acid levels do not come down to normal levels with a low dose of the medication. There are side effects to taking this medication, including joint pain, nausea, and muscle pain.

• Allopurinol. This is the most commonly used medication for reducing uric acid levels. Like Febuxostat, it decreases the amount of uric acid produced in the body. Many doctors start out with a low dose of the medication and increase it until the uric acid levels return to normal. This means having your blood checked periodically to see how the medication is working. There are side effects to this medication as well, such as stomach problems and a rash. These side effects are usually transitory and go away after you have taken the drug for a period of time. Rarely, severe allergic reactions can occur when giving this drug so you need to inform your doctor if you do not feel well when taking the medication.

•   Probenecid.   This is a drug that acts to make the kidneys excrete uric acid at a faster rate.   It is often taken with antibiotics as the combination makes the probenecid work better. As with other drugs for reducing uric acid levels, you need to be aware of side effects, such as headaches, stomach problems, rash, kidney stones, nausea, and vomiting. Tell your doctor if you are experiencing any of these side effects.

• Pegloticase. This is a medication that is used as a last resort after other medications fail to reduce the uric acid levels in your blood stream. It works faster than most of the other medications and is said to be used for "refractory chronic gout" in which the uric acid levels remain elevated despite taking the usual medications for this condition. There are side effects to taking this medication, including nausea, vomiting, constipation, chest pain, bruising, reactions related to giving the medication by IV, and a flare-up of gout. If you have any of these side effects, talk to your doctor about switching to another medication.

Self-Care for Gout

You can reduce the symptoms of gout by simply taking better care of yourself. This will reduce the side effects you could have experienced if you took medications for gout. Self-care involves eating a healthier diet, losing weight, and getting regular exercise. These things alone can decrease the chances of another attack of gout and will also work toward decreasing your risk of heart disease, which commonly goes along with having gout.

Dietary Goals

A healthy diet can go a long way toward decreasing your risk of heart disease and gout. It involves eating a diet that is high in fruits, vegetables, whole grain products, and proteins derived not from meat but from legumes and nuts. Low fat dairy products are also acceptable. The foods you want to stay away from include any type of processed food and foods that are high in refined carbohydrates.

These are the foods you'll want to stock up on if you want to decrease your uric acid levels and decrease your risk of heart disease:

- Coffee
- Vitamin C-containing foods, such as oranges, limes, grapefruit, and lemons (supplements are also acceptable)

- Water, which flushes uric acid out of the kidneys

- Low sugar fruits that have a low glycemic index (the glycemic index a measurement of how fast the sugars in the fruit are absorbed in the bloodstream)

- Vegetables of any type

- Oils that are plant-based, such as sunflower oil, canola oil, and olive oil

- Whole grain products, such as brown rice and whole wheat bread

- Low fat dairy products, such as skim milk, cottage cheese, and low fat yogurt

- Cherries, which lower uric acid levels

These are the foods you'll want to avoid if you are trying to keep your uric acid level down. They contain a lot of purines, which are the main triggers for gouty arthritis:

- Alcohol. You will want to drink no more than 2 alcoholic beverages per day if you are a man and less than one alcoholic beverage per day if you are a woman.

- Beverages that are high in sugar, such as sugar-containing sodas and energy drinks high in sugar.

- Lobster and shrimp, which contain a great deal of purines in them.

- Organ meats, including liver, sweetbreads, and tongue.

- Any type of red meat, such as steaks, hamburgers, and roast beef.

- Refined foods that are high in carbohydrates. They contain foods that will increase uric acid levels.

Physical Activity to reduce Gouty Attacks

Any type of physical activity you do will decrease your weight and will limit the amount of gouty attacks you have. Exercise that causes weight loss will decrease the level of uric acid in your system and can decrease your risk of cardiovascular side effects, such as heart attacks, strokes, and peripheral vascular disease. These things seem to go along with having gout. You need to start by exercising gradually, working your way up to 30 minutes of aerobic activity per day on most days of the week. If you are not used to exercising and might already be at risk for developing heart disease, you need to talk to your doctor about having an exercise stress test, which can measure your ability to exercise. This will insure to a reasonable degree that your heart will withstand the rigors of exercise.

While it isn't easy to start an exercise program, the rewards are great. Not only will you have a reduction in gouty arthritis attacks but you will decrease your risk for heart disease. Try to choose a physical activity that you enjoy so you will be able to stick to it longer and will enjoy it more.

Complications of Gout

While having an attack of gout is bad enough, there are complications of gout that make it a much more serious disease. Common complications of having gout include the following:

• Advanced gout. This occurs when you don't adequately treat a gouty attack. When you have untreated gout, you may develop tophi, which are collections of uric acid crystals that build up in the tissues, particularly around the joints. The elbows, your Achilles tendon, feet, hands, and fingers are the main areas where tophi develop. While they are unsightly, they generally do not cause pain and can resolve with medications used to treat elevated uric acid levels. In rare cases, tophi can swell and become sore, especially when you are having an attack of acute gouty arthritis.

• Recurrent gout. This is when you have elevated uric acid levels and have many cases of gouty arthritis within a year. Medications to control elevated uric acid levels can reduce the incidence of recurrent gout. Most of these medications are fairly well tolerated and can be taken chronically to avoid additional attacks of gouty arthritis. If you don't treat an attack of gouty arthritis, the joints can erode and can be destroyed by uric acid crystals.

• Kidney stones. Uric acid can build up in the kidneys that normally secrete uric acid in the urine. This causes crystals of uric acid that can be extremely painful. Fortunately, medications that reduce the production of uric acid will also decrease your chances of having uric acid kidney stones. If you have kidney stones from elevated uric acid levels, you will often have flank pain and blood in the urine—both telltale signs that you have uric acid kidney stones.

Alternative Medications for Gouty Arthritis

If you have tried medications for gouty arthritis and they fail to work, there are many alternative medical choices for gouty arthritis. These alternative medications shouldn't be taken lightly as they can interact with other medications you are taking for gout or other medical conditions. Speak to your doctor before you start a regimen of alternative medications for gout. These remedies are often not studied very well in scientific studies so it isn't completely clear whether they actually work to prevent attacks of gouty arthritis.

Here are some alternative medications and foods that can decrease uric acid levels in your system:

• Vitamin C. You can take vitamin C supplements that will decrease the chances that you will have gouty arthritis. While vitamin C supplements will lower uric acid levels, there is no evidence that it will actually prevent an attack of gouty arthritis. More research needs to be done to see if this is a viable option for you. On the good side, there is no harm in taking vitamin C supplements, so they are worth a try.

• Coffee. There have been actual research studies showing a benefit to drinking coffee if you have elevated uric acid levels. It turns out that both decaffeinated coffee and caffeinated coffee will decrease the levels of uric acid in your system. The main problem with drinking coffee for gouty arthritis is that scientists do not know the mechanism of action of coffee in the reduction of gouty arthritis attacks.

• Cherries. You can lower your level of uric acid simply be eating cherries. Research studies have shown a connection between cherry consumption and the development of gouty arthritis. You can eat cherries directly from the supermarket or you can drink cherry extract to reduce uric acid levels. There are also dried supplements that are made from cherries. While cherries are completely safe to take, you should talk to your doctor about using cherries as a way of decreasing your levels of uric acid.

There are other alternative medical techniques that can decrease your uric acid levels and can perhaps decrease the risk of having gouty arthritis. This can include meditation and relaxation techniques. They work to decrease the perception of pain in those patients who have gouty arthritis and are completely safe to do.

Prevention of Gout

The best way to deal with gout is to prevent an attack from happening in the first place. Fortunately, there are medications you can take that will essentially keep you from attacks of gouty arthritis. If you have extremely painful attacks of gouty arthritis or several attacks per year, you may wish to consider taking one of the following medications:

• Drugs that block the production of uric acid. This includes drugs such as allopurinol, which is marketed as Zyloprim, Lopurin, and Aloprim, and Uloric, which is the brand name for febuxostat. Both of these drugs are helpful in decreasing the production of uric acids. By decreasing uric acid levels, your chances of having an attack are extremely low. There are side effects you'll want to consider. Allopurinol can cause decreased blood cell counts and rashes, while febuxostat can cause decreased effectiveness of the liver, nausea, vomiting, and a rash.

•   Drugs that enhance the removal of uric acid. This includes Probalan, which is the brand name for probenecid. This drug enhances the ability of the kidneys to get rid of uric acid from your system. This drug has the effect of decreasing uric acid levels in the bloodstream, shunting it towards the kidneys where it can be effectively excreted through the urine. Common side effects of probenecid are kidney stones, stomach pains, and rashes.

When you are feeling better and have no symptoms of gouty arthritis, you can follow a special diet that can help reduce the incidence of gouty arthritis. Some dietary measures you might want to undertake include the following:

• Try to attain a normal body weight. This means selecting smaller portion sizes that will keep you from eating too many calories. When you lose weight, you will have lower levels of uric acid in your system and fewer attacks of gouty arthritis. Try not to fast or lose weight too quickly because this can actually make your system worse.

• Decrease the amount of poultry, fish, and meat you are eating. These kinds of foods raise purine levels and can precipitate an attack of gouty arthritis. You may not need to swear off these foods altogether but instead eat fewer portions of these meats per week. Aim for no more than 3 servings of poultry, fish, or meat per week.

• Use low fat dairy products as protein sources. As you won't be getting protein from meat, you'll need another source of protein. Low fat dairy products are high in protein and yet will not cause gouty arthritis unlike meat sources of protein.

• Stay away from alcohol. There is research evidence that excessive alcohol intake can precipitate an attack of gouty arthritis. The link is especially true of beer drinking. Seek medical advice when deciding how much alcohol you should be drinking. A reasonable goal is to have less than 2 drinks per day (for men) and less than 1 drink per day (for women).

• Keep your intake of fluid high. Gout is made worse under circumstances of low hydration. In order to avoid this, you will want to drink as much fluids as possible. You can choose just about any beverage (except alcohol) but plain water is considered the best.

Exercises for Gout

When you are suffering from an attack of gouty arthritis, exercise would seem like the last thing you would want to do. In actuality, however, exercise can be good for gout. When you don't exercise, you can set up a cycle that makes the disease worse. When you have an attack, your joints may be too sore to exercise vigorously but, when you are feeling better, exercise can increase the flexibility of the joints and can strengthen your muscles.

Exercise during gouty attacks may need to be limited to range of motion exercises that will help the arthritis heal and will keep your joints from stiffening up. Exercise you engage in when your attack has diminished will help you increase your bone mass, and will improve the health of your muscles and joints. All it takes is a program of moderate exercise to decrease the risk of gout. Moderate aerobic exercise will also decrease your risk of heart disease. Anaerobic exercise, such as weight lifting and using weight machines can build muscle mass and will enhance your bone density. When you are able to exercise on a regular basis, you will have better energy and an increase in strength. Be sure to follow a healthy diet at the same time as the combination will decrease your chances of having a flare-up of your gout.

The following are exercises that will decrease your chances of having an attack of gouty arthritis and will improve your cardiovascular health. You can do aerobic exercises that increase your heart rate and respiratory rate (which improves cardiovascular function) or exercises the build muscle mass (anaerobic exercise). Doing both types of exercise (anaerobic and aerobic) will decrease your gout symptoms and will help you maintain better health.

Be sure to talk to your doctor before starting any type of exercise activities, especially if you are at risk for heart disease. You may wish to undergo an exercise treadmill test that will check to see if your heart is healthy enough for exercise.

Aerobic Exercise

You'll want to select some low impact exercises that will maximize your cardiovascular system and improve the function of your lungs. Aerobic exercises involve doing things like brisk walking, swimming, jogging, and bicycling. They will improve your heart health and will increase the strength of the muscles in your legs.

Begin your aerobic exercise program by exercising about ten minutes per day. As your exercise fitness increases, you can build up to exercising 30-45 minutes each day for most days of the week (4-5 days should be enough.

One of the best aerobic exercises you can do is swimming. You can do lap swimming in a large pool or engage in water aerobics, which can increase your flexibility and cardiovascular fitness without putting undue stress on your joints. Swimming is especially good because it doesn't put extra stress on your joints.

Start by swimming about 10 minutes per day and work your way up to swimming 30 to 45 minutes per day. You don't have to swim aggressively. Mild to moderate swimming exercises are sufficient to enhance your cardiovascular function and will improve the muscle strength supporting the joints.

You can also do stretching exercises. Stretching exercises can help increase the flexibility of your upper and lower body. Start by stretching the muscles of your arms and shoulders. Put your arms by your sides and do a series of shoulder rolls in order to stretch the muscles of the shoulder. Roll the shoulder muscles in a forward direction for about half a minute and repeat by rolling the shoulders in a backward direction for another half a minute.

You should also exercise your wrists. You can do this by making a fist with your hands and rolling your wrists in all directions for several minutes. While gout rarely affects the wrists, stretching all the muscles of the body is important.

You can also stretch the muscles of your hamstrings and back. You can do this by sitting on the floor. Put your legs in front of you and then try to reach forward until you reach your toes. This stretches the hamstrings and your back at the same time. Hold the pose for about 15 seconds and repeat several times per day to stretch these areas of your body.

Natural Supplements for Gout

If you don't want to take prescription medications for gout but still want some relief of your gouty symptoms, you can turn to natural supplements to decrease your gouty symptoms. There are many natural substances that will lower your uric acid levels, enhance your immune system, and decrease the amount of inflammation in your body.

Before starting to take supplements for gout, seek your doctor's advice about which supplements you should take. Not all supplements are backed by scientific research but are instead folklore medications that have been used for centuries. Even though most are safe, they can interact with medications you are already taking so your doctor should know when you've started a supplement.

Here are some supplements you might want to try (with your doctor's permission):

• Omega 3 fatty acids. Omega 3 fatty acids can be gotten through eating cold water fish like tuna, salmon, halibut, and sardines. You can also take a fish oil supplement. These contain docosahexaenoic acid (DHA) and eicosapentaenoic acid (EPA)—both of which are especially good omega 3 fatty acids.

• Gamma-Linolenic Acid. This is also referred to as GLA. Gamma-linolenic acid is a type of omega 6 fatty acid that can decrease the symptoms of gout. The best sources of GLA include borage oil, evening primrose oil, and black current seed oil. They decrease the inflammation seen in gouty arthritis. They make gamma-linolenic acid supplements that you can purchase at any good health food store. Take them as directed or ask your doctor how much you should take.

•   Methylsulfonylmethane (MSM). This is an organic sulfur-based compound that increases the rate of connective tissue formation. According to the American Academy of Pain Management, MSM can help reduce the pain of gouty arthritis. The best source of MSM is an MSM supplement taken in amounts approaching 3,000 milligrams twice daily. This will decrease the levels of inflammation in your body and will decrease your gout-related pain.

• Folic Acid. Folic acid is also referred to as folate. It has been found to be helpful in people suffering from gout. By taking a folic acid supplement, you can cause the degradation of homocysteine in your system. Homocysteine is often elevated in those who have elevated levels of uric acid. Folic acid supplements are easy to take and can be taken alone or as part of a multivitamin. •Vitamin C. Vitamin C is a good all-around vitamin to take for better health. For gout sufferers, however, vitamin C is especially helpful. If you don't already have gout but have elevated uric acid levels, vitamin C can prevent the onset of gout. If you already have gout, vitamin C can decrease the number of gouty attacks you have per year. You can take a vitamin C supplement or increase the amount of vitamin C in your diet by eating fresh fruits and vegetables. • Ermiao wan. This is an herb found in Traditional Chinese Medicine. It has been used for many centuries for the treatment of gout. It is especially good for gout because it has fewer side effects when compared to prescription anti-gout medications. As it is an uncommon herb, you may wish to talk to an herbalist before using this supplement for your gouty symptoms. • Other herbs. There are other herbs that you can try to decrease uric acid levels and decrease the frequency of gouty attacks. Some of these herbs include bromelain, Devil's claw, and turmeric. They all have anti-inflammatory properties and will help in enhancing your immune system. Try making a tea out of any one of these herbs or take them as a packaged supplement. You can buy the supplements at your local health food store or can get them through a qualified herbalist.

• Cherries. As mentioned, cherries seem to have anti-gout effects. They contain anthocyanines that have anti-inflammatory properties. They also reduce the level of uric acid in the body and decrease the frequency of gouty arthritis attacks. In one research study on cherries and gout (published in 2012), eating about ten cherries per day can decrease the risk of gouty arthritis attacks by 50 percent. Similar findings were found when subjects with gout took a tablespoon of tart cherry extract. A tablespoon of tart cherry extract is the same a eating 45-60 cherries twice daily.

Dealing with a Loved One with Gout

Not only does gout affect the individual with elevated uric acid levels, but it can affect their loved ones as well. Living with someone who has gout means dealing with the chronic pain your loved one has and coping with their inability to be productive around the house or at work.

Because as many as 84 percent of gout sufferers will have an attack in the next 3 years after their first attack, loved ones must be prepared for recurrences and must help the gout sufferer with their diet and exercise program necessary to prevent further attacks. During an attack, the entire household may be under stress as the pain is so intense, it affects all areas of the individual's life.

Living with a person with gout is a lifelong process. The exacerbations of gout can be very trying on the whole family, and can affect the daily activities of both the gout sufferer and his or her entire family. As the individual ages, the frequency of gouty arthritis tends to increase so that you may find yourself dealing with gout on a regular basis. This can be trying on any relationship.

Gout Resources

If you are dealing with gout, it is important to remember that you are not alone and that you have resources to help you get through the disease with decreased pain and better overall function. One great resource is your rheumatologist. A rheumatologist is a specialist in joint diseases such as gouty arthritis. They can help establish the diagnosis of gout in the beginning stages of the disease and can help the gout sufferer lower uric acid levels and decrease the frequency of gouty attacks.

While you can see a regular internist for the treatment of gout, a rheumatologist has special expertise in this area and may be more helpful when it comes to the latest treatment guidelines and treatments that ordinary doctors have no knowledge of. If you believe you have gout, ask for a referral to see a rheumatologist for further diagnosis and management.

Another resource for gout is Gout Awareness Day. Gout Awareness Day occurs each year on May 22nd. It provides a forum for gout sufferers to remember what they know about the disease and to learn all they can about how it is treated and how gouty arthritis can be prevented.

Out of Gout Awareness day came a program known as "Let's Speak Gout", which is co-sponsored by Takeda Pharmaceuticals and the Arthritis Foundation. The goal of this program is to get the word out about gout and its effects on its sufferers. It can also help you find local resources that will steer you toward the best rheumatologists and the best treatments for the disease.

Through "Let's Speak Out", you can learn ways to work with your rheumatologist to improve your communication about your gout symptoms. You can learn ways to advocate for yourself when you see the doctor, resources for tracking gouty symptoms and attacks of gouty arthritis, and learn about ways you can decrease your uric acid levels so you won't have as many gouty arthritis attacks.

The Arthritis Foundation can be another resource for people with gout. They have access to local resources in your area and sponsor research efforts aimed toward finding better ways to prevent and control gout. Check with your local chapter of the Arthritis Foundation or contact them at 1-404-872-7100. They have a website that allows you to find local chapters of the Arthritis Foundation and a toll-free helpline, which is 1-844-577-HELP.

Misinformation about Gout

Gout is a real and serious disease that affects millions of people throughout the world. Over the years, however, there has been a lot of misinformation about gout that interfere with the gout sufferer from getting the treatment they need to help their disease.

Contrary to what many people think, gout is not a disease of slovenly men who drink too much alcohol and eat too much red meat. Gout can affect anyone with any lifestyle habits and can have a hereditary component that doesn't have anything to do with lifestyle or obesity.

Because of the misinformation about gout, many people feel too embarrassed to seek the medical attention they need to control their symptoms. One study out of the Auckland University looked at 114 different articles on gout stemming from 2010 to 2015 in the US and the UK. While most of the articles came from the tabloid news, some came from respected periodicals, such as the Washington Post, The Guardian, and The New York times.

According to the study, people with gout are believed to have an embarrassing condition brought on by poor lifestyle habits such as eating foods that are too rich and drinking too much alcohol. This prevented people from seeking the proper medical treatment they needed in order to control their disease.

Of the 114 articles they looked at, 72 of the articles indicated that gout was caused mainly by excesses in eating and drinking. In one article out of the Wall Street Journal, writers indicated that gout was present only in slovenly people who drink large amounts of alcohol and indulge in eating too much red meat. Only 46 of the articles studied actually noted that gout can be caused by biological conditions that are out of a person's control, such as kidney problems and heredity.

Many of the articles referred to gout as being a socially embarrassing disease and a third of all articles lacked the seriousness that gout deserves. Joking about gout in these types of magazines and newspapers only prevents those who believe they are suffering from the disease from getting the care they need to feel better and to live healthy, active lives.

Less than 50 percent of the articles studied actually talked about strategies to manage gout and those that did focused solely on the dietary measures one could take to counteract the effects of gout. Only 42 of the articles talked about medical treatments for gout, such as febuxostat and allopurinol.

Ideally, gout should be referred to as much more than having a swelling of the toes. Articles talking about the facts of gout should note that gout cannot be helped in some cases and that things like heredity and kidney disease play just as much of a role in getting the disease as lifestyle habits.

Even though high purine foods can contribute to getting gout, about 66 percent of uric acid is naturally made by the body and doesn't come from the food we eat at all. Even so, cutting back on purine-containing foods can help people with high uric acid levels avoid flare-ups of the disease. Gout can also be precipitated by taking certain drugs for other medical conditions. It is not an embarrassing disease and doesn't mean that you aren't taking care of yourself.

Contrary to many of the misinformation-based articles out there, gout can be managed not only by lifestyle changes but by medications that lower uric acid levels. Drugs can be taken to both decrease the uric acid levels in the body, and to decrease the inflammation and pain once a gouty attack starts. These drugs can also improve kidney excretion of uric acid in order to decrease the uric acid levels in the symptom and to prevent uric acid crystals from forming kidney stones.

Another problem with misinformation about gout is that many people believe that they will be chastised by their doctor about their eating habits and won't be taken seriously. Instead of getting the help they need to reduce their symptoms, they instead choose to tolerate the pain and aren't getting proper care. They are also missing out on the important information they need to have in order to prevent another attack of gout from occurring.

To set the matters straight, it should be noted that gout is not just a matter of overindulgence in rich foods and alcohol. There are many other factors that go into getting gout that have nothing to do with eating and drinking habits. The newspaper and magazine articles are wrong in telling people that having gout is all their fault.

Side Effects from Gout Drugs

Allopurinol (Zyloprim) is perhaps the most common medication used in the management of elevated uric acid levels. Unfortunately, it has a serious side effect. It can cause a relatively rare, yet possibly life-threatening skin rash. This side effect seems to occur at a higher risk among people of African descent or Asian descent. This has recently come out in an article published in Seminars in Arthritis and Rehabilitation.

The 2 main skin reactions associated with taking allopurinol are toxic epidermal necrolysis (TEN) and Stevens-Johnson syndrome (SJS). Besides a skin rash, both of these conditions involve blistering of the skin and mucus membranes, a rash that includes most of the body, and flu-like symptoms. Besides damage to the skin, the internal organs can be damaged.

While SJS and TEN are two skin conditions, many doctors believe they have the same basis (origin) but show up differently in different individuals. Both are potentially life-threatening and can lead to death from organ failure if not properly treated in a hospital setting.

According to the latest research, people who are of Asian descent have a twelve-fold increase in the risk of these two skin reactions, while people of African descent have a five-fold risk for developing these conditions.

This doesn't mean that they shouldn't use the drug; it just means that they need to be monitored more carefully and warned of the possibility that this type of side effect may occur. There are treatments for both these conditions and a chance that the person's life can be saved if they seek medical attention as soon as they notice a rash.

The risk of toxic epidermal necrolysis and Steven's-Johnson syndrome is usually the highest in the first 6 months of starting the drug. If a reaction has not begun to occur by this time, there is practically no chance that it will later occur. Even so, people taking the drug should be aware of this possible side effect.

One study was done on the risk of SJS and TEN in patients who took allopurinol. They looked at hospitalization records of as many as eight million people. Of these individuals, about 600 cases of SJS or TEN were identified.

When the researchers looked more carefully, they found that those who developed the rash were more likely to be Asian or African in descent. This doesn't mean that it didn't show up in Caucasians and other ethnicities but the risk of these diseases in Caucasians was much less in this population. In fact, 29 percent of all cases of TEN and SJS occurred in Caucasians.

The overall risk of developing these skin reactions to allopurinol was calculated to be about 1 out of every 4000 Caucasians, 1 out of every 740 people of African descent, and 1 out of every 340 people of Asian descent. The risk in Hispanics was believed to be similar to the risk in Caucasians.

The researchers further revealed that those people who had an HLA type (human lymphocyte allele) of B 5801 had the highest risk of having a negative skin reaction when taking allopurinol. This genetic makeup occurs to a higher degree in African Americans and Asian Americans. This isn't to say that everyone should be tested for the HLA type as this would be cost prohibitive and the incidence of these skin reactions is extremely rare.

On the other hand, the American College of Rheumatology (ACR) indicated in 2012 that Asian Americans with gout should be tested for this HLA type before giving them allopurinol for their gout. The blood test for HLA typing costs only about $150, which isn't a high price to pay among Asian Americans who have SJS or TENS to such a high degree after taking allopurinol. If the patient tests positive for the allele, they are often placed on another drug to lower uric acid levels, such as febuxostat or probenecid.

Those who take allopurinol tend not to take it for a short period of time. As gout is a chronic, lifelong condition, the need for allopurinol is likely to last a person's lifetime. Taking allopurinol can lower uric acid levels and can decrease the frequency of attacks of gouty arthritis.

The idea to take the drug safely and on a regular basis so that the symptoms don't come back. Besides its risk of causing SJS and TEN, allopurinol is relatively safe and has few side effects. It is generally preferable to take the drug and risk side effects than it is to suffer through an attack of gouty arthritis that may come on a recurrent basis.

For those that do develop SJS or TEN from taking allopurinol, about a third of all patients die from their disease. Those patients that don't die from these conditions often have extensive eye damage and kidney problems for the rest of their lives.

The study mentioned above raises concerns about anyone of Asian or African descent taking allopurinol. Hopefully, if high risk patients are screened for the HLA 5801 and given other medications to lower their uric acid levels, then the risk of developing SJS or TEN goes down considerably. If you are Asian American or African American and are already taking allopurinol, see your doctor about getting tested for the allele and possibly consider switching to another drug.

Case Study on Gout

The following is a case study on an individual who was basically healthy before coming down with gout:

The patient, whose name was Scott, was a former football player and former wrestler who was healthy with the exception of knee problems that resulted in three separate knee operations. He was used to pain from surgery and from his sports activities but never experienced a pain as severe as the one he had when he developed gouty arthritis. He knew a great deal about gout as his father had the condition for the last 20 years. Because of his family history, he knew he was at a greater risk for the disease and watched his weight, exercising regularly and avoiding foods that trigger gout.

Even so, he developed a severe pain in his right great toe that was so painful he couldn't tolerate having bed sheets touching his toe. The toe was swollen and red by the time he presented to his internist for evaluation. He was placed on indomethacin and referred to a rheumatologist. The rheumatologist drew blood for uric acid and found it to be elevated. He also took a sterile syringe and aspirated some of the joint fluid in the great toe. Under the microscope, the classic findings of uric acid crystals could be detected. The indomethacin was continued and Scott had resolution of his symptoms after a couple of weeks.

After that, he went back to the rheumatologist and it was decided that he be started on allopurinol (Zyloprim) to reduce his uric acid levels. As he wasn't of African or Asian descent, he wasn't tested for the HLA 5801 allele. He was also instructed to follow a low purine diet similar to the one his father was on. Scott took the allopurinol for six months but stopped it as he was having no symptoms. Three months later, he developed symptoms of gouty arthritis occurring again in his right great toe. After a trip to the rheumatologist to get back on indomethacin, Scott decided that having another attack of gouty arthritis wasn't worth it. As it was clear that he needed to be on something to lower his uric acid level in order to avoid further attacks, he started back on the allopurinol and takes it regularly. He has not had another attack of gouty arthritis since restarting the allopurinol.

Summary

Gout is an inflammatory condition involving crystals of uric acid developing in the joints. Risk factors for the disease includes having a history of gout in the family, kidney problems, obesity, and a high purine diet. While gout does not cause cardiovascular disease, they carry the same risk factors and those with gout should be screened for heart disease as well.

Uric acid levels can be elevated for many years before a person gets an attack. No one knows exactly what precipitates an attack of gouty arthritis but it could be related to eating a food that triggers the consolidation of uric acid crystals in the joint or it could be an injury to the joint that inflames the joint, resulting in gouty arthritis.

There is no cure for gout but there are medications and lifestyle changes that contribute to getting gout. Many people with recurrent attacks of gouty arthritis need to take medications to reduce their overall uric acid levels.

Gouty pain is not something you need to deal with. There are medications that can effectively get rid of the inflammation so that the flare-up can be managed. It usually takes about 10 days before the symptoms go down. It is not a good idea to take a uric acid-lowering medication while having an acute attack of gouty arthritis as this can make the pain worse. The time to take a uric acid-lowering medication is when there are no longer any signs or symptoms of inflammation in the joints.

While many people take allopurinol to lower uric acid levels, there are other medications available, especially for those of African and Asian descent, who are at a high risk of developing serious skin conditions such as toxic epidermal necrolysis (TEN) and Steven's Johnson syndrome (SJS)—both of which can be life threatening. There is a blood test that can be taken that will determine if you are at risk for these side effects while taking allopurinol.

At the first sign of pain and redness in a joint, you need to see your doctor and be evaluated for gout. After the attack of gout has resolved, you can take medications to make sure you don't get another attack.

Your Reviews are greatly appreciated, and your gout experiences help others cope with their own. Please do share your experiences, and help others deal with gout.

action, application or preparation, to any person reading or following the information in this book. References are provided for informational purposes only and do not constitute endorsement of any websites or other sources. Readers should be aware that the websites listed in this book may change.

This guide is not intended to be any type of Medical advice. ALL individuals must consult their Doctors first and should always receive their meal plans from a qualified practitioner. . This book is not intended to heal, or cure anyone from any kind of illness, or disease. This book is for educational, and reference purposes only.

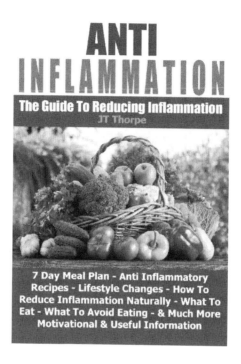

Anti Inflammation

The Guide to Reducing Inflammation

7 Day Meal Plan – Anti Inflammatory Recipes – Lifestyle Changes –
How To Reduce Inflammation Naturally – What To Eat – What To
Avoid Eating - & Much More Motivational & Useful Information

JT Thorpe

This Book contains information that is intended to help the readers be better informed consumers of health care. It is presented as general advice on health care. Always consult your doctor for your individual needs. This book is not intended to be a substitute for the medical advice of a licensed physician. The reader should consult with their doctor in any matters relating to his/her health. No part of this Book may be reproduced or transmitted in any form or by any means, electronic or mechanical, including photocopying, recording or by any information storage and retrieval system, without written permission from the author.

So what is inflammation?

I am going to go out on a limb and guess that you have a negative impression of the word inflammation. After all, we are constantly bombarded with advertisements for expensive medications that promise to reduce inflammation (at the expense of some nasty side effects.) We never hear anything positive about the word. So it may surprise you to learn that inflammation is actually a complex biological response that is crucial to our health and well-being. This is because inflammation is meant to protect the body's tissues against harmful stimuli such as pathogens, harmful bacteria and irritants. When the body is functioning normally and a pathogen invades our body, our white blood cells cause our bodies to heat up and essentially burn out these intruders. An example of useful inflammation is the body's response to the common cold; when the viral infectious disease enters our body, our noses and throats become inflamed in an effort to drive the cold out. This means that your immune system is working correctly.

So why has inflammation become such a dirty word? Well, it is because sometimes the body gets confused. In the presence of certain diseases, such as arthritis, gout and even some forms of cancer, the body will trigger an inflammatory response when there are actually no pathogens to fight off. In doing so, the body's immune system actually causes damage to the body rather than fixing anything. The white blood cells release chemicals into blood and tissue which increase blood flow, causing redness, warmth, and occasionally swelling and pain. Chronic inflammation can lead to sever tissue damage over time.

However, before you reach for the pill bottle, it might again surprise you to know that in nearly all cases, the best way to fight inflammation is actually through your diet. Modern diets are rife with foods that can cause and exacerbate inflammation, simply because the body does not quite know what to do with them. There are also many key lifestyle changes that you can make in order to feel better and stop your body's immune system from spinning out of control.

This guide is designed to take you through the building blocks of your diet and show which foods are causing you pain and why. Then you are going to learn not only which foods can start you on the path to recovery, but also many delicious ways to prepare them! So let's dive right in and start feeling better today.

Signs of Inflammation:

(Often, only a few symptoms will present themselves in any given case.)

- Redness
- Joint pain and/or stiffness
- Swelling of joints
- Joints feel hot to the touch
- Flu-like symptoms such as fever, chills, fatigue, headaches, muscle stiffness, loss of appetite.

In order to be diagnosed, it is best to visit your doctor if you experience any of these systems. In order to diagnose you with an inflammatory disease, your doctor will have to examine not only your symptoms, but also your medical history. The doctor will likely run a series of tests, including blood tests and X-rays.

Examples of Inflammatory Diseases

Inflammation has become a source of great worry for many healthcare professionals, nutritionists and those who work in the food industry. Various forms of arthritis are connected to inflammation, such as rheumatoid arthritis, psoriatic arthritis, and gouty arthritis (often known simply as gout.) Inflammation may also be a symptom and/or cause in diseases and disorders such as hay fever, periodontitis, diabetes and cardiovascular disease.

But the truth is, inflammation is just a symptom. It is not a condition in itself. Instead, damaging inflammation is the result of the damaging things we do to our body every day. Unhealthy foods, too much emotional stress and repeated physical injuries will all lead to an increase in inflammation and much higher chance of contracting one of the diseases listed above. In many cases, inflammation just comes along with the territory of the disease, but for a few, inflammation can be the cause of developing a new condition.

And the rate of inflammatory diseases is on the rise. In recent years, 65 percent of arthritis diagnoses were for people under the age of 65. Young people are twice as likely as their parents to develop this painful and sometimes debilitating disease. Rates of diabetes have increased 49 percent in 10 years, and inflammatory reactions to high levels of glucose increase the chances of suffering diabetes related blindness, heart disease and cancer. New studies are revealing that the damage inflammation inflicts on artery walls in the heart are just as impactful as harmful cholesterol.

Chronic inflammation is both painful and dangerous. If you suffer from chronic inflammation it is critical that you seek to reduce the factors in your life that are causing it. Your body will thank you for it.

How to Reduce Inflammation

Inflammation reduction is not an exact science. Fortunately, thousands of doctors, dieticians and other healthcare or food professionals have been working hard for years researching new and improved methods of reducing inflammation. These methods can be divided into three different sections: diet, lifestyle and medication.

Diet

(Note: It is important to talk to your doctor any time you are considering making major changes in your diet)

Nutrition is a major determinate of inflammation – and often the easiest thing for most people to change. Many healthcare professionals and dieticians are now harshly criticizing our modern diets as the leading factor in the increased rate of painful inflammation. Fortunately, a great deal of research has gone into testing the effects of different foods and diets, and most experts agree that the basic principles of the Mediterranean diet - diet low in processed foods and saturated fat and rich in fruits, vegetables, fish, nuts and beans – are excellent guidelines. To understand why, lets break down food into its three components – fat, protein and carbohydrates – and study how these components either contribute or combat inflammation.

Fat

First of all, fat is not the enemy. Fat is a crucial part of the human diet and without it we cannot live. A typical recommendation is to receive 30 percent of your daily calories from fat. However, not all fats are created equal, and modern diets often contain high levels of certain types of fats that our bodies have difficulty processing. These include saturated fat and trans-fatty acids. Saturated fats generally come from animal products like red meat and cheese. They trigger inflammation in the body's fat tissues which both increases the likelihood of developing heart disease and worsens inflammation from arthritis. Trans-fatty acids are found in popular processed food items like doughnuts, stick margarines and cookies. Trans fats are the absolute worst fats for your body and trigger systemic inflammation, particularly in women.

On the flip side, unsaturated fats are known as the healthy fats – as long as they are consumed in moderation as part of an overall balanced diet. Unsaturated fats contain essential fatty acids Omega-3 and Omega-6, which work together in the body to reduce risk of heart, liver and brain disease, among other maladies. However, consuming too much of either of these fatty acids can also trigger inflammation. Foods rich in good unsaturated fats include salmon, vegetable oils, nuts and eggs.

Protein

Nearly all of the foods discussed in the last section are also rich in protein – another extremely crucial part of a human diet. Most experts agree that about 30 percent of your daily calories should come from proteins. However, like with fats, not all proteins are created equal. The basic principles of the Mediterranean diet suggest that our diets should be full of fish and plant-based proteins, rather than proteins from red meat and dairy products. Lean meats like chicken and turkey have their place within the diet too, but studies suggest that fish, nuts and beans are the healthiest sources of protein available and the least likely to trigger an inflammatory response.

Carbohydrates

The main role of carbohydrates is to produce glucose, which the body converts into energy. Typically, you want to receive 40 percent of your calories from carbohydrates, which rounds out to 100 percent, after the 30 percent fat and 30 percent protein. While most people think of breads and pastas when they think of carbs, the truth is that we get carbohydrates from many different foods, such as grains, sweets, fruits, vegetables and dairy products. The only main food group without many carbohydrates is meat. Carbohydrate sources vary wildly when it comes to nutritional value and health benefits, and their power to either reduce or increase inflammation can be calculated based on their glycemic index.

The glycemic index measures the impact that foods have on our blood sugar levels. Low-glycemic carbohydrates help to reduce inflammation, whereas high-glycemic carbs can make it worse. Low-glycemic carbohydrate sources are general unrefined and unprocessed - whole grains, such as barley, oats and brown rice, fresh fruits and vegetables, and low-fat milk and unsweetened yogurt. High-glycemic carbohydrates come from processed foods and foods with high amounts of sugar, such as white flour, instant rice, soft drinks, candy, potatoes and doughnuts.

Herbs and Spices

Herbs and spices do not fit into any of the three categories above, but some of them can also have a major impact on inflammation. Many herbs and spices contain antioxidants, vitamins and minerals that are all beneficial to our health. Oxidation is closely related to inflammation, so herbs and spices containing anti-oxidants are especially effective in fighting the good fight. Chili peppers contain a compound called dihydrocapsiate which boosts your body's capacity to burn fat. Herbs and spices also add flavor to food without adding calories - this reduces the amount of sodium, fat and/or sugar we feel compelled to add to our dishes.

Topping the list of the best spices for reducing inflammation are ginger, rosemary, turmeric, cloves, basil, oregano, garlic, cilantro, cayenne pepper, sage, thyme and everyone's favorite – cinnamon. There are so many delicious ways to use each of these spices that there is really no excuse not to give them a try. Within weeks you could find yourself not only experiencing less inflammation, but also shedding unwanted pounds since you are no longer loading your food with fat and salt to make it taste better!

Beverages

Everything you put in your mouth can have a role in fighting or causing inflammation and drink are certainly no exception. Health care professional and dieticians have long struggled with counseling people to watch what they drink, as it is even easier to drink excessive amounts of calories than it is to eat them. After all, one Frozen Mocha Coffee Coolatta from Dunkin Donuts can have up to 990 calories! That's more than three McDonalds cheeseburgers, and chances are you could drink the coffee in a third of the time it would take you to eat those cheeseburgers. Therefore, it is easy to drink excessive quantities of inflammation-causing beverages without realizing how much you are consuming. A good rule of thumb is to avoid any drinks that either high in sugar or high in sugar substitutes. Chemical sweeteners and flavorings of any kind are very irritating to your gut.

Coffee is a tricky subject. Experts go back and forth on whether or not coffee is good for inflammation or causes inflammation. On the one hand, coffee contains anti-oxidants, which as we know from the previous section on herbs and spices, can be very useful in fighting inflammation. On the other hand, studies have found a correlation between moderate-to-high coffee consumption and an increase in inflammation. As we wait for more studies to clear up this confusion, there is no need to quit coffee cold-turkey, but if you drink massive amounts of coffee each day, it might be good to moderate yourself a little, and see if you feel any better for it.

The rules for alcohol are very similar to those for coffee. Small amounts of alcohol – particularly red wine – have been shown to have health benefits and reduce stress, which is good for fighting inflammation. However, alcohol metabolizes as pure sugar in the body and too many drinks will irritate your gut and cause bacteria to pass through the intestinal lining. So enjoy responsibly!

Finally, what beverages are good for fighting inflammation? As always, you need to be drinking enough water per day. Staying hydrated is often the number one way to improve your immediate and long-term health and comfort. Another excellent beverage to add into your daily routine is green tea. Green tea has long been touted for its fat-burning potential and it is loaded with antioxidants. However, remember not to load your green tea with sugar – that will most likely cancel out its benefits. Instead, try adding a splash of real lemon juice to bring out the tea's refreshing flavor.

Putting It All Together

All this information is well and good, but it doesn't tell you how to construct an actual eating plan that will help you to reduce inflammation and give you relief from pain and swelling. What you need now is a comprehensive list of food to avoid whenever possible, and a guide to the best way to enjoy healthy foods that will improve your quality of life. The good news is that a diet designed to reduce inflammation does not have to be restrictive. If you are thinking to yourself that from now on eating will be a chore and bore, you're wrong! That being said, we eat a lot of junk in our modern diet – a lot of foods our body was not meant to process in the quantities we eat them. Next you will find a comprehensive list of foods to limit or avoid from your diet if you want to stop inflammation before it starts.

Foods to Limit and/or Avoid in Your Diet

Note that this is not necessarily a list of foods to cut out of your diet completely. For many people, facing the prospect of never again indulging in their favorite foods is a deal-breaker. You might start out with the best of intentions, draw up a list of "banned" foods in your household, and start holding yourself to your new diet with military discipline. Then the first time you walk past that box of Oreos in the store, or see your favorite pasta dish on the menu, you will cave and decide that this is too hard and you are just going to forget about the whole thing.

But the truth is, simple becoming more conscious about your food choices and reaching for the healthy, anti-inflammatory foods nine times out of ten is still going to make a world of difference! So when you are perusing this list and you see a food that you just know you cannot give up completely, tell yourself that you are going to start viewing that food as a rare treat. Maybe you will tell yourself that you are going to start having only ONE doughnut every other Sunday. Or you will have a cheeseburger only when you go to the neighbor's grill-out. Chances are, after a few months, your favorite treats will even start to taste better because a) they will be a novelty, b) you won't feel guilty about eating them, and c) best of all – you will feel so much better inside!

With that being said, here is a list of foods that unfortunately promote inflammation.

Fatty, red meats (steak and burgers)

Processed meats (hot dogs, deli meats, pepperoni)

Soda (regular and sugar-free)

White potatoes

Processed/fried vegetables (French fries, onion rings)

Fruit juices (high sugar content)

Foods with artificial dyes or flavorings

White breads and pastas

Canned/preserved fruits (this includes jams, jellies and marmalades)

Mono-sodium glutamate (MSG, a popular ingredient in many fast food dishes, Asian cooking and salad dressings)

High-gluten foods

Stick margerine

Farmed fish

Corn, soybean, and sunflower oils

High sodium foods

So What to Eat Instead?

If looking at the list above made you despair, it's time to snap out of it! Yes, there are many delicious things on that list – but there are even more delicious things on this next list! Our modern diets have become depending on heavily processed, sugared foods and it is making us very unhealthy. Isn't it time to nip that in the bud and discover how food can be both tasty and nourishing? Here is a list of foods that ought to be part of your diet.

Fish (Wild salmon, anchovies, mackerel, herring, sardines and trout)

Chances are you've heard this one before. That is because fish has been shown to be one of the absolute best sources of inflammation-fighting omega-3 fatty acids. Experts suggest consuming three to four ounces of fish at least twice a week, and some arthritis experts swear by the power of eating fish daily to reduce painful swelling. Unfortunately, not everyone is fond of fish. If you just cannot bring yourself to eat any of these varieties of fish, there are fish oil supplements you can take that are available in just about any grocery or drug store.

Nuts and Seeds

This should be a cause for celebration! Nuts are packed with both monounsaturated fat and vitamin B-6 – and both have been shown to fight inflammation. The best nuts to munch on are almonds, pistachios, walnuts and pine nuts, and the serving recommendation amounts to about a handful and a half (1.5 ounces) per day.

Colorful fruits and vegetables

The benefits of fresh fruits and vegetables is well-known, but the most colorful ones have the highest levels of antioxidants. Dark, leafy greens like kale and spinach, brilliant red and blue cherries and berries, and bright citrus fruits should all be welcome additions to your diet – and to your table. Impress your guests with salads that are almost too beautiful to eat!

Olive Oil

Okay this might seem like a strange one – how can oil be one of the best things for you? Well, olive oil beats out other vegetable oils because it is loaded with heart healthy fats, and because olive oil is less refined and processed than other oils, meaning that it retains more of its nutrients. And if you can get your hands on them, avocado and walnut oil can be just as healthy, if not healthier than olive oil.

Beans

Beans are an excellent source of protein with little fat content, and their high fiber content is great for the gut. Our serving suggestion is two or more cups a week.

Whole grains are far superior to their white bread counterpart. They contain more fiber which has been linked to lower blood levels of an inflammatory protein. However, whole grains do often contain high levels of gluten, which has been linked to inflammation in some people, so you should discuss any negative reactions to whole grains with your doctor who can help you determine whether or not you have an intolerance to the gluten.

Lean meats and poultry

Shellfish (crab, shrimp, mussels)

Egg whites

Whole milk dairy and cheese

Dark chocolate

Yes! You do not have to give up chocolate. Dark chocolate is full of antioxidants.

The next few pages, you will find a seven day meal plan guide, and recipes. These are just a few ideas, for breakfast, lunch, dinner, and snacks. These are just ideas, that you, and your doctors can go over, and see if they are good choices for your personal diet.

SUNDAY	Apple and ginger whole wheat muffins	Turkey Chili	Pan-Seared Salmon on baby arugula	Baked garlic shrimp
MONDAY	Baked pears with blue cheese and walnuts	Warm spinach and mushroom salad	Sweet Potato Black Bean Burgers	Fennel, apple and celery salad
TUESDAY	Fish tacos	Lebanese tabbouleh salad	Italian stuffed red peppers	Greek yoghurt with strawberries
WEDNESDAY	Coconut quinoa porridge with ginger and dates	Grilled chicken and kale Caesar salad in a spinach wrap	Drunken Mussels	Roasted mixed nuts
THURSDAY	Raspberry smoothies	Shrimp and vegetable soup	Parmesan-crusted pork chops	Celery and carrot sticks with hummus
FRIDAY	Spinach and mushroom frittata	Eggplant parmesan sandwiches on whole-grain	Pecan rosemary baked tilapia	Baked apples with cinnamon and ginger

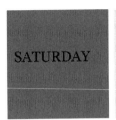SATURDAY	Apple cinnamon and blueberry oatmeal	Tuna salad sandwiches	Grilled balsamic and garlic flank steak	Baked kale chips

Now of course comes the question of how to start incorporating all these healthy foods into our diets. That's why we have provided a menu outlining seven full days of anti-inflammatory meals – breakfast, lunch, snack and dinner. This is the part that should be fun – learn new cooking techniques, dazzle your friends and family with your newfound culinary skills and feel better in the process. With this template, you can mix and match meals for a month, keeping things fresh and never boring.

Note: Recipes for several of the foods listed in this guide can be found below.

BREAKFAST   LUNCH   DINNER   SNACK

SUNDAY   Apple and ginger - whole wheat muffins - Turkey Chili -   Pan-Seared Salmon on baby arugula   - Baked garlic shrimp

MONDAY   Baked pears with blue cheese and walnuts - Warm spinach and mushroom salad -   Sweet Potato Black Bean Burgers -   Fennel, apple and celery salad

TUESDAY   Fish tacos - Lebanese tabbouleh salad - Italian stuffed red peppers -   Greek yogurt with strawberries

WEDNESDAY   Coconut quinoa porridge with ginger and dates   - Grilled chicken and kale Caesar salad in a spinach wrap   - Drunken Mussels   -   Roasted mixed nuts

THURSDAY   Raspberry smoothies - Shrimp   and vegetable soup - Parmesan-crusted pork chops - Celery and carrot sticks with hummus

FRIDAY Spinach and mushroom frittata - Eggplant parmesan sandwiches on whole-grain ciabatta - Pecan rosemary baked tilapia- Baked apples with cinnamon and ginger

SATURDAY Apple cinnamon and blueberry oatmeal- Tuna salad sandwiches Grilled - balsamic and garlic flank steak - Baked kale chips

Recipes

Spinach and Mushroom Frittata

Ingredients

- 2 tbs butter
- 3 cloves minced garlic
- 1/2 cup sliced onion
- 1 cup sliced mushrooms
- 2 cups chopped spinach
- 6 eggs
- 1/2 tsp salt
- Dash pepper
- 1/2 cup grated parmesan cheese

Directions

Melt the butter in a skillet.

Add garlic, onions and mushrooms. Cook until onions are translucent.

Add spinach and sautee for two minutes.

Beat eggs, salt and pepper together in a small bowl and then pour over mixture in skillet, stirring to combine.

Cook eggs until they are almost set but still moist on top. (About four minutes)

Sprinkle on parmesan cheese and place skillet in oven.

Broil for four minutes or until eggs are set and cheese is lightly browned

Coconut Quinoa Porridge with Ginger and Dates

Ingredients

- 1 cup quinoa
- 1 1/2 cups coconut milk
- 1 cup water
- 1-inch piece sliced fresh ginger
- 1 tablespoon brown sugar
- Pinch of salt
- 1/2 cup chopped dates
- 1/4 cup chopped crystallized ginger

Directions

Rinse the quinoa three times, draining in a fine-mesh sieve after each rinse.

Put the quinoa, coconut milk, water, fresh ginger and salt in a medium saucepan. Bring to a boil over medium heat, then reduce the heat to low and simmer, stirring occasionally until the quinoa is tender and most of the liquid has been absorbed (About 20 minutes.)

Remove from the heat and discard the ginger slices.

Drizzle with the remaining coconut milk and top with the chopped dates and crystallized ginger. Serve warm.

Shrimp and vegetable soup

Ingredients

- 2 tbs olive oil
- 1 chopped onion
- 1 chopped carrot
- 1 chopped fennel bulb (keep the fronds)
- 2 tbs tomato paste
- 1 lb peeled and deveined medium shrimp
- 2 28-oz bottles clam juice
- 1 14.5-oz can diced tomatoes
- salt and black pepper

Directions

Heat the oil in a large saucepan over medium heat.

Add onion, carrot, and chopped fennel and cook until softened (6 to 8 minutes.)

Stir in the tomato paste.

Add the shrimp, clam juice, tomatoes and their juices, and 1½ cups water to the saucepan.

Season with salt and pepper.

Simmer until the shrimp are opaque, about 2 minutes.

Sprinkle with the fennel fronds and serve.

Drunken Mussels

Ingredients

- 2 tbs butter
- 4 cloves garlic, minced
- 1/2 tsp red pepper flakes, or to taste
- 1 lemon, zested
- 2 cups white wine
- freshly ground black pepper
- 2 lbs mussels, cleaned and debearded
- 1 cup chopped parsley
- 2 slices grilled bread
- 2 lemon wedges for garnish

Directions

Melt butter in a large stock pot over medium heat.

Add garlic and cook for 30 seconds.

Season with red pepper flakes and lemon zest, stirring for about 45 seconds.

Quickly pour in wine into the pan and season with black pepper.

Bring sauce to a boil, stir in mussels, and cover immediately.

Shake pot and let boil for 1 minute.

Stir mussels, replace cover, and let boil for 2 more minutes. The shells will begin to open.

Stir in parsley, cover pot, and cook until all shells are open, 1 to 3 minutes.

Serve with grilled bread and lemon wedge.

Pecan Rosemary Baked Tilapia

Ingredients

- 4 4-oz tilapia fillets
- 2 tsp fresh rosemary
- 1 egg white
- 1/2 tsp packed brown sugar
- Pinch cayenne pepper
- Dash of salt
- 1 1/2 tsp olive oil
- 1/3 cup raw pecans
- 1/3 cup breadcrumbs

Directions

In a small baking dish, stir together pecans, breadcrumbs, brown sugar, salt and cayenne pepper.

Add the olive oil and toss to coat the pecan mixture.

Bake at 350 degrees F until the pecan mixture is light golden brown, 7 to 8 minutes.

Increase the heat to 400 degrees F. Coat a large glass baking dish with cooking spray.

In a shallow dish, whisk the egg white. Working with one tilapia at a time, dip the fish in the egg white and then the pecan mixture, lightly coating each side.

Place the fillets in the prepared baking dish.

Press the remaining pecan mixture into the top of the tilapia fillets.

Bake until the tilapia is just cooked through, about 10 minutes. Serve.

Fennel, Apple and Celery Salad

Ingredients

1/4 cup plus 2 tbs lemon juice

1 tbs extra-virgin olive oil

Salt and black pepper

2 large apples, julienned

1 medium head fennel, cored and thinly sliced

3 large ribs celery, sliced

1/2 cup cilantro leaves, roughly chopped

Directions

In a large bowl, combine the lemon juice, olive oil, salt and pepper. Add the apples, fennel, celery and cilantro. Toss until well combined. Taste and adjust seasonings.

Tips for adjusting to a new diet

Change is never easy, and it is especially difficult when it comes to our diets. Many people start out strong with a new eating plan, full of motivation to change their habits for the better. But motivation can be fleeting. Sometimes all it takes is one rough day for us to turn back to the comfort of familiar tastes. Here are a handful of tips to make it easier

•   Give your palate time to adjust by gradually replacing the unhealthy junk with better foods. For example, replace your white toast in the mornings with oatmeal. Replace a hamburger with a helping of salmon. Even these small changes can have a big impact, and once you realize how much better you are feeling, you will be more inclined to make other changes. Slowly but surely you will replace the bad with the good.

• Avoid focusing on what you "cannot" or "should not" eat. Instead, focus on shifting the balance of your diet to healthier foods. If there is something you love to eat even though it exacerbates your inflammation, set aside specific days to treat yourself with a small portion.

• Plan meals and snacks in advance to avoid unhealthy impulse eating. Take time each week to map out a menu and to prepare foods in advance and refrigerate or freeze them.

• Research restaurants before you go out to eat to see if they have dishes that comply with your new dietary requirements.

The Best (and Healthiest) Ways to Indulge

No one should have to give up on dessert completely and any diet that tries to make you is most likely doomed to fail. However, since an excess of sugar has been shown time and time again to be a major promotor of inflammation, you need to be clever when choosing a sweet to end your meal. Here are a few desserts that are perfect for people looking to clear up their inflammation.

Mexican Hot Chocolate

This treat combines dark chocolate, almond milk and cinnamon – all foods that have been mentioned so far as being friendly to our bodies. The dark chocolate and cinnamon contain powerful antioxidants, while the almond milk contains healthy fats. Heat 4 ½ cups of almond milk in a saucepan to just below a simmer. Then add 5 ounces of finely chopped dark chocolate and stir continuously until the chocolate has melted. Stir in a dash of cinnamon and serve warm.

Grilled fruit

Okay, this one might sound a little strange, but just try it out. Slice up some pineapples, bananas, pears or apples and throw them on the grill. Grilling reduces the water content of the fruit so that each bite packs more flavor. It can also caramelize the natural sugars, giving you that candy taste without refined sugars.

Banana "Ice Cream" with Cinnamon and Walnuts

At this point, you are probably sensing a pattern – replacing simple carbohydrates with complex ones. Regular ice cream is high in white sugar. Bananas contain natural fruit sugar, along with fiber and potassium. For this dessert, blend chunks of frozen banana with almond milk until it is the consistency of ice cream. Sprinkle on some chopped walnuts and cinnamon.

Baked Ricotta with Berries

Ricotta is a soft, mild-flavored cheese often used in Italian cooking. When baked, it can serve as a delicious substitute for cheesecake. Simply mix whole milk ricotta with one egg, two tablespoons of brown sugar and half a teaspoon of vanilla extra. Bake at 350 degrees for 20 to 25 minutes or until nicely golden. Remove from the oven and let sit for two minutes, then serve with berries and a light drizzle of honey (optional).

The Lifestyle Changes That Will Reduce Inflammation

(Note: It is important to talk to your doctor any time you are considering making major changes in your exercise regimen and lifestyle. Sometimes major changes can shock your system in unexpected ways.)

Now that you have a clearer understanding of how your day-to-day diet can affect inflammation, it is time to discuss some of the overall lifestyle changes you can make that will lead to a healthier, pain-free you. Just as our modern diets tend to fill our bodies with junk, our modern lifestyles often prevent us from engaging in healthy habits. Americans spend more on healthcare now than at any other point in time, and some experts warn that younger generations are going to be the first generations in which the children are less healthy than their parents. It is incredibly easy in this day and age to eat too much, never exercise and burn out from stress. All of these things can and will lead to increased inflammation.

Changing your lifestyle is not an easy thing to do. It requires motivation and discipline in equal measure. If you are not motivated, you will never be able to discipline yourself. If you have no discipline, your motivation will keep you setting goals that you never actually work towards, and that will only increase your stress levels.

In order to start, you need to tell yourself that there is nothing more important right now than becoming healthier. It is all too easy to tell ourselves that we simply don't have time to exercise, or that our stress is a necessary and integral part of getting ahead in our careers and relationships. But the truth is that you either learn how to integrate healthy living into your routine now or you pay the consequences later. Will your spouse, children, friends, boss thank you when you are laid up in the hospital, unable to socialize or work, because you let your chronic inflammation destroy your body? What does it matter that you worked hard if you never have the chance to reap the rewards?

Our bodies are amazing things and they allow us to do so much. It is time to give back to your body by making changes for the healthier. By following this next set of guidelines, you are giving the future back to yourself.

Lose Weight

Obesity has officially become an epidemic in America, with nearly 36 percent of adults qualifying as obese based on their body mass index measurements. Nearly two-thirds of American adults qualify as overweight. If you are one of the few who are within a healthy weight, this section will not apply to you, but if you are carrying around even an extra 10 to 20 pounds of fat, you are at a higher risk for developing chronic inflammation.

How does that work? Basically, fat cells create chemical signals that lead to chronic inflammation, especially when you regularly overeat and overindulge in sugar. These chemical signals interfere with the function of insulin in our bodies, aggravating insulin resistance and worsening the symptoms of type 2 diabetes. Our fat cells expand when we gain weight, and causes them to give out even more signals that aggravate inflammation. When we lose weight, the fat cells are able to shrink back to their normal capacity, and stop sending out as many chemical signals. Of course, losing weight is easier said than done and keeping weight off is especially hard. Reports show that the majority of people who lose a significant amount of weight will gain it back (and sometimes more) within a year. The reason for this is that people are not willing to put in the effort to lose weight in a healthy way. They go on binge diets, essentially starving themselves for a short period to shed pounds as quickly as possible. The problem with this is that often the weight you lose in that short period of time is water weight. When you start to eat regularly again, you gain it back very quickly. People also turn to supplements that promise get-thin-quick solutions. Spoiler alert: just about every one of these solutions is completely bogus. Yes, there are extreme cases when doctors will prescribe extreme measures and medicines to help their patients lose weight, but that is almost always only when they patient has a specific medical reason why they are unable to lose weight normally. I'm afraid that the rest of us are just going to have to buckle down and commit to a new lifestyle in which the calories we expend are more than or equal to the calories we take in. This is how weight is lost. And the most effective way to lose weight is through changing your diet. It is much easier to not eat 200 calories than it is to spend an hour sweating in the gym to burn off those 200 calories. The diet plan described earlier is full of healthy foods, so if you are paying attention to eating only anti-inflammatory foods you are already on the right path. Now what you need to do is track your calories to make sure you are not eating too much. There are plenty of great websites and mobile apps that make tracking calories easy and even fun. SparkPeople and MyFitnessPal allow you to log your meals, calculate calories and even calculate the balance of fat, protein and carbohydrates in your diet. They also have online forums where you can meet other people who are on the same mission to lose weight and get healthy. Finally, these sites have tons of delicious new recipes every day.

It's going to take time. Experts say that a healthy amount of weight to lose is no more than two pounds per week, and even that involves a 7,000 calories deficit. It is going to be hard and discouraging at times, but you need to constantly remind yourself that even if you cannot see the progress, you are making your body healthier. And chances are, if you are suffering painful inflammation as a result of being overweight, you will begin to feel better even before you notice a difference in your waistline.

Reduce Blood Sugar

This suggestion has its own section because while it is linked with losing weight, reducing blood sugar is its own battle. It is entirely possible to reduce overall calories without cutting out simple carbohydrates – much more difficult but possible. Foods like white flour, refined sugar and high fructose corn syrup dump massive amounts of junk into your body that your body was just not made to deal with. Chronically high levels of blood sugar can eventually lead to developing type 2 diabetes. That is why it is so important to stick to the diet plans and food guides from section one, and replace the simple carbohydrates with good, complex carbs found in healthier foods.

It is also important to ask your doctor about your blood sugar levels. Your doctor might have more radical suggestions for reducing these levels if they are high enough to be of immediate concern.

Physical Activity

I know I said before that diet was a much more effective way of losing weight than exercise. But exercise is also very important and regular physical activity has benefits beyond the simple gain or loss of pounds. The reason I am using the phrase physical activity instead of exercise is that most people tend to think of exercise as a chore – going to the gym, slogging away on the treadmill, lunges, weight-lifting and more. And while that is certainly a type of physical activity, there are so many more fun ways to keep yourself moving throughout the day. The average American sits 10 hours a day. All this sitting around greatly increases your chances of being overweight, but it also allows your muscles to atrophy to the point where any type of physical activity becomes dangerous because your body is no longer capable of handling it. So one of the first changes you need to make if you are one of these chronic sitters is to find ways to get up and move every hour. If you work a desk job, take a short stroll to the next office or cubicle to talk to a coworker rather than sending an email. Get up and get a drink of water. Take your lunch outside rather than eating at your desk. If you are sitting because you want to watch TV or read a book, find something physical to do that will not distract you from the story – stretching, walking or jogging in place. And more importantly, do something fun with your body! Take a dance class, go swimming at the YMCA, play a game of catch with your family and friends. If you have a dog, they are probably dying to get walked more. Visit your neighbors. The bottom line is that you need to get up and move, in any way you can make that happen. Now of course, this does not mean discounting higher intensity exercise entirely. It is important to build up your muscles – people with more muscle mass burn more calories on average than people with less. But you don't have to torture yourself on the treadmill for hours if you really hate it. Instead, many doctors are recommending HIIT – High Intensity Interval Training. HIIT involves performing high intensity exercises for short periods of time, followed by a brief period of rest, and then doing it again. Many HIIT routines last no longer than half an hour, so they can easily be incorporated into your daily routine. You don't even have to shell out for a gym membership – many HIIT routines are available on DVD or streaming sites like Amazon.com.

Of course, you may have heard that exercise can also increase inflammation. However, depending on the context, this exercise-induced inflammation is not necessarily a bad thing. Remember – inflammation just means that your body's immune system is chugging away. When you do physical activity, you are essentially breaking down your muscles in order to let them rebuild themselves bigger and stronger. Therefore, exercise can lead to inflammation, but it will be acute inflammation – the helpful kind that gets in, repairs the tissue and gets out. Of course acute inflammation can sometimes turn into chronic inflammation if you do not give yourself proper recovery time. This is why it is important to incorporate rest days into your exercise routine, and, as always, consult with your doctor before starting a new regimen.

The bottom line is – it's time to get moving! If you are sitting on your butt all day, you are not going to be feeling your best.

Quit Smoking Just as with dieting and exercising, quitting smoking comes with a vast variety of health benefits. There are few single things you can do to increase your quality of life and likely lengthen it than by quitting smoking, because according to the World Health Organization, Smoking is the single largest preventable cause of disease and premature death. But why does it make such a big difference when it comes to inflammation? Smoking greatly increases the response of the immune system to vascular injuries – injuries caused by some form of physical trauma. By triggering this overresponse, smoking increases levels of inflammatory markers. This means that smoking is a major factor in not only chronic lung disease, but also heart disease and stroke. Research on women who quit smoking revealed extraordinary results – the women showed major reduction of inflammatory biomarkers within a few weeks!

Of course I realize that "quit smoking" is much, much easier said than done. Quitting any addiction is a grueling process and nicotine withdrawal is especially nasty. That is why it is important to seek the help of professionals as well as family and friends. There are more helpful products than ever before designed to helping you kick the habit – gums, patches, medications and even cigarette alternatives such as vapors and ecigarettes. And the good news is, if you can stick with it for just a little bit, you should start feeling less inflammation within weeks!

Avoid Repetitive Motions

Repetitive motion injuries are injuries to the tissue that can be caused by any number of repeated motions, such as typing, throwing a ball or scrubbing the floor. The injuries are some of the most common in the United States. Repetitive motion injuries most frequently occur in the tendons and the bursae (small sacs within the body that provide cushioning to joints), and cause inflammation, known as tendinitis and bursitis. While this inflammation generally starts off as acute – attempting to heal the damaged tendons and/or bursae – if you ignore the warning signs and continue to injure the inflamed area, it can turn into chronic inflammation. These injuries can become quite serious and even land you in the hospital if you manage to pick up an infection.

People sometimes do ignore these injuries for too long because they try to shrug it off as just the normal pain of day-to-day living, but it is very important to take care of your tendons and bursae, especially when you are younger. If you notice that an area of your body in which you engage in repetitive motion is feeling inflamed, seek medical help to determine what can be done. Doctors may ask you to rest the area or wear protective gear such as wrist braces.

Reduce Stress

This is another one of those things that seems like a no-brainer, but if you look at the state of the average American lifestyle you will see stresses piling upon stresses with no chance for relief in sight. Surveys from the last few years have shown that stress levels are consistently rising – and it is not just affecting adults. A 2011 study showed that nearly a third of children exhibiting some type of physical symptom that is linked to stress. 86 percent of children said that their parents' stress levels had an effect on them.

Stress triggers inflammation due to cortisol. Cortisol is a steroid hormone produced from cholesterol and it plays several very important roles within our bodies. One of these roles has traditionally been called the "fight or flight response." Stress is a survival mechanism. When a person is faced with a stressor, his or her adrenals secrete cortisol which immediately floods the body with glucose, as an emergency supply of energy to stimulate the muscles. The cortisol blocks insulin production, preventing the glucose from being stored. It also narrows the arteries while at the same time making blood pump faster. Traditionally, the person would then engage in fight or flight – he or she would defend themselves against the attacker or run away from it. After the situation was resolved, the hormone levels would return to normal, and the body would go on relatively unscathed. However, in our modern world, the source of our stress is rarely a physical attacker. Instead, things like bills, tests, deadlines, significant others, children and more cause us to stress out – and in our fast-paced lifestyles, we rarely have time to de-stress and allow our hormone levels to normalize. This extra cortisol wreaks all kinds of havoc on our bodies. It creates imbalances in blood sugar, leading to weight gain and type 2 diabetes, gastrointestinal problems and cardiovascular problems – all of which are linked to inflammation.

Fortunately, stress is not just a given. It is something we can prevent and solve with enough patience, forethought and dedication. By employing methods to reduce the stress in our lives, and the lives of those around us, we can allow our hormones to take a break.

Preventing Stress

As the saying goes, an ounce of prevention is worth a pound of cure. Americans experience an incredible amount of unnecessary stress, often simply due to not knowing how to handle conflict and disappointment. In order to prevent our stress levels from rising while we are on the job, with family, or on the road, we must practice several different methods of keeping ourselves calm. One of the first steps is simply to identify the sources of stress in our lives. Maybe you are getting into the same fight with your spouse every day. Maybe your morning commute is always full of frustration. Maybe you are constantly procrastinating at work and then having to pull all-nighters to finish big projects. You alone know where the stress is coming from in your life.

Some people find it helpful to use a stress journal, giving them a chance to analyze both the source and how they responded to it. And actually it is crucial to examine your reactions to stress and how you cope, because many people using coping methods that might seem like they help, but they are in fact short-term solutions that are causing more long-term problems in the end. Examples include binge eating, smoking and drinking – all of which have already been mentioned as sources of inflammation. Once you realize that you are employing one of these flawed coping methods, you can brainstorm alternatives. The next time you feel yourself reaching for the chips after a bad day at work, take a walk outside instead. Or read a book or paint a picture. There are thousands of productive, calming things you can be doing.

Communication skills are critical when it comes to avoiding stress. When we feel that we are not being heard, or when we have a tendency to lash out at others that causes us incredible guilt after the fact, we really get that cortisol flowing. Practice things like saying "no" – so many people take on too much in their day-to-day life because they are too afraid to say no. Then, after you have committed yourself to something you do not have the time, energy or desire to do, you might engage in passive aggressive behavior, which can trigger a chain reaction of hurt feelings and retaliation. That kind of drama is absolutely useless. Also, learn how to constructively address arguments and conflicts, using statements that do not place blame and seeking out the help of an impartial mediator if you know that a conversation is going to incite strong emotions and anxiety. Learn to practice forgiveness. Keeping negative emotions bottled up for any reason will only exacerbate those emotions and increase stress. All of these things and more are ways that we can winnow out the badness in our lives. Practicing these will solve a whole host of problems besides inflammation. Managing Existing Stress Of course some amount of stress is completely unavoidable. In many ways stress is what defines us as human beings because it keeps us moving, keeps us working, keeps us trying. And a good dose of that cortisol is not inherently a bad thing – unless we never manage to get it to leave our system. Once you have removed the unnecessary stressors from your life and you are left with the immoveable ones, it is time to figure out how to relax. This does not seem like it should be such a hard thing to do, relaxing, but unfortunately it can be easy to screw up relaxation time and end up with more stress – and inflammation – than you started out with. Picking vacations that don't match with your interests, spending more time with the family that is causing you stress, engaging in those behaviors mentioned in the previous section that will only increase stress in the long run – these are all things that people do and then wonder why they do not feel as refreshed as they thought they would. Managing stress actually involves delving deeply into your psyche and figuring out what you uniquely would like to be doing with your time that you are not doing. That is why these next few suggestions are not for everyone. That being said, they are tried and true methods that thousands of people do use every day to manage their cortisol output and so there must be something to them. If you are a person who simply does not know how to relax, go ahead and try a few. See what you like and don't like, and when you find that thing that makes you feel calm, make time for it. Do not feel guilty about taking care of yourself.

Stretch into Some Yoga Is there anyone who hasn't heard of the health benefits of yoga? Besides helping with weight loss, building muscle tone and increasing flexibility, yoga involves deep breathing and fluid motions that slow down the heart rate and allow you to focus completely on your body and how it works for you. We spend so much of our time ignoring our body's real needs and we also ignore all the ways that our bodies are incredibly well-crafted to keep us alive. Yoga can be practiced alone, but often the social aspect of taking a class can be just as rewarding as the exercise itself. If you feel anxious because you have never taken a class before, look for a beginner's session and remind yourself that everyone there is too focused on themselves to even notice what you are doing. Or, take a friend with you so that you have someone to laugh with if you are feeling ridiculous. Plus, chances are high you will run into several people who are trying out yoga for the same reason you are – because they are experiencing too much anxiety in their lives. Open yourself up to an experience that has helped people clear their mind and cleanse their soul for hundreds of thousands of years.

Get a Massage

This is another one of those things that doctors keep touting the positives of. We carry a lot of our stress physically – in our backs, shoulders and necks. If you experience chronic muscle pain and there is no apparent physical reason, there is a good chance that your anxiety is transferring itself to your physical body as a desperate cry for help. Our bodies and our minds should not be thought of separately – they are intertwined and affect each other in a myriad of ways. That is why masseuses reveal that often people cry while they are receiving a massage. As all that tension drains out of them, they experience a cathartic release accompanied by tears. Humans are social creatures and we are not meant to go any length of time without some sort of friendly touch. The touch of a masseuse – or even a friend of family member – in the course of a mission to make you feel good could be just the thing to lift you out of chronic stress.

Take a Bath

Much like the massage, a hot bath targets the muscles that receive our stress and helps them to relax. And there is something pretty magical about taking an hour of your day to just feel good. It makes a big difference in both the short term and the long run. You can enjoy your bath simply, or add in all your accessories – bath bombs, Epsom salts, scented candles. Read a book, listen to music, enjoy a cup of tea or (one!) glass of wine. Lay back and imagine that there is nothing in the world except for you and that hot water caressing your skin.

Work in a Garden There is a (slightly cynical) Chinese saying that goes "A Chinese Saying – If you want to be happy for an hour, get drunk – if you want to be happy for a day, get married – if you want to be happy for life, plant a garden." Planting a garden is creating something – bringing something living into this world that will never talk back to you or borrow your car. Gardening allows you to gently work your body and exposes you to sunlight. Be sure to apply sunblock in order to avoid UV damage, and then feel free to soak in that feel-good vitamin D. The repetitive tasks give you a chance to regulate your breathing – much like yoga – and offer a chance for meditative reflection. Finally, planting a garden is all about hope – the hope that you will reap your flowers, or vegetable, or herbs. It gives you a chance to step out of yourself and focus on nurturing something else. And in a strange twist, this is an act of healing yourself. Now, gardening is not for everyone. For some it is just another chore, and chores are definitely not a good way of relieving stress. But you will never know if a garden can be a positive thing for you unless you try. So if you have never tried, start small, with one plant or some window boxes. See how you feel when things start blooming.

Pet Some Puppies

In a similar fashion to planting a garden, the joy of interacting with an animal that does not make demands of us beyond our love. Dogs especially have been bred over the years to be in tune with human emotions and behavior, and many times they can tell when we are anxious or depressed even before we can. In addition, animals are the perfect sounding board for our problems because they listen with absolutely no judgement. Often, people are not looking for someone who professes to be able to solve their problems. They just want someone to listen and sympathize. Animals will listen and in return they will give you love.

Owning a pet is a form of informal therapy every day. However, not everyone is in the position to care for an animal and if that's the case, owning a pet will cause you more stress than before. However, there are hundreds of thousands of animal shelters all over the country. Sign up as a volunteer and receive a little therapy time while also providing an invaluable service. And if you really feel that you need more help than that, many therapists provide professional animal-assisted therapy services.

Laugh

It's hopelessly cliché but that doesn't make it any less true – laughter really is the best medicine. Laughter stimulates your heart, lungs and muscles, floods your body with endorphins and allows your stress response to activate and then immediately relax, which soothes the tension in your body. Laughing with a friend or loved one can be especially rewarding because it allows you to bond over feeling good. So treat yourself to a night at the comedy club with a few buddies, or snuggle up next to a special someone and pop in a funny movie.

Join a Book Club

Reading is often a solitary activity, and curling up alone with a good book really hits the spot for some, but for others it can lead to feelings of loneliness. After all, when you really like something, you want to tell other people about it. If you feel that you have real insight into the inner workings of a particular character, you want to know if others felt the same way. Book clubs offer a chance to make new friends, have your opinion validated and also to just keep working out our brains. One of the secrets to keeping your brain healthy is to never stop learning. Book clubs are all the fun of learning without the stress of tests and term papers.

Seek Professional Help

Sometimes we really just can't go it alone. The key is to recognize when our stress is having a severe impact on our lives, and having the courage to take steps to relieve it. Psychiatrists exist to improve the quality of life of their clients. There is no shame in asking for help, and chances are that if you suffer greatly from stress, your loved ones are suffering because of your stress too. They will thank you for doing what you can to make yourself healthier.

Get Enough Sleep

A lack of sleep can dramatically weaken your immune system. In fact, losing just a few hours of sleep in the space of a single night can trigger tissue-damaging inflammation. This is especially problematic for women, but both sexes should practice healthy, regular sleeping habits. This means establishing a routine in which you go to bed and wake up at the same time every day. Experts say that six hours is the absolute minimum amount of sleep you should be receiving, and most recommend between seven and nine hours per night, though this depends on several factors including age. If you have difficulty sleeping for any reason, you should seek medical help. Avoid eating or drinking caffeine before bedtime and practice calming rituals such as reading a book or meditating before bed. Wake up well rested and feeling better than ever!

Medication Of course, sometimes you can try all the wholesome, natural methods in the book and they still won't be able to solve 100 percent of your inflammation problems. The human body can be a strange thing, and no two people operate in exactly the same way. All of the suggestions made previously have merit to them, not just in solving inflammation, but generally when it comes to health and well-being. It is worth trying many of them even if they do not completely solve your problem. But eventually it might come time to speak to your doctor about taking medication to suppress inflammatory responses. These are called nonsteroidal anti-inflammatory drugs (NSAIDs) and they generally work by decreasing the swelling and pain that result from the inflammation. Some NSAIDs can be found over-the-counter while others require a prescription. Since modern medicine comes out with new drugs regularly, I will not suggest any specific medications here, but rather encourage you to consult with your doctor about your specific problems and needs. Be open and honest about your diet and lifestyle when doing so, and don't be surprised if your doctor suggests trying several of the methods of diet and lifestyle changed mentioned in this document. Let your doctor guide you through the process of choosing the right drugs for you.

Conclusion

I sincerely hope that this guide has given you some insight into the causes, symptoms and potential solutions for your inflammation. It is one of the most common causes of pain and illness and while doctors are doing everything they can, a lot of it is really up to each individual to manage their health. When you neglect your body, your body will act out. When you put things in your body that it was not meant to process, you will reap what you sow. Thankfully, living a lifestyle coordinated to fight inflammation does not have to be awful – it can be delicious, fun and relaxing if you do it right! If this guide has you feeling overwhelmed, remember that you do not have to try everything at once. You do not have to change your diet in one day. Instead, start small and grow into a new routine gradually. I predict that when you start feeling better, you will want to keep going, keep doing more for your body.

Good luck!

We thank you, and value your comments, and reviews for this book. Please share your experience with others, so they may benefit from your knowledge on the subject. Your experiences, and thoughts, can help benefit those struggling with diabetes, more than you could possibly imagine. Placing your ideas, and experiences in the review section of this book, will make it seen by others, who will benefit from your help. 5 minutes of your time, can help change someone's life for the better. Thank you.

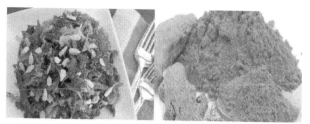

ANTI - INFLAMMATORY

COOKBOOK

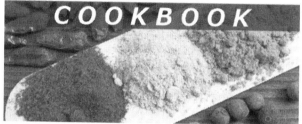

50
Slow Cooker Recipes With
Anti - Inflammatory
Ingredients

GREAT FOR GOUT RELIEF!

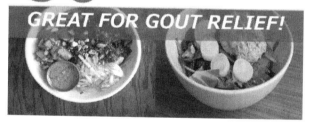

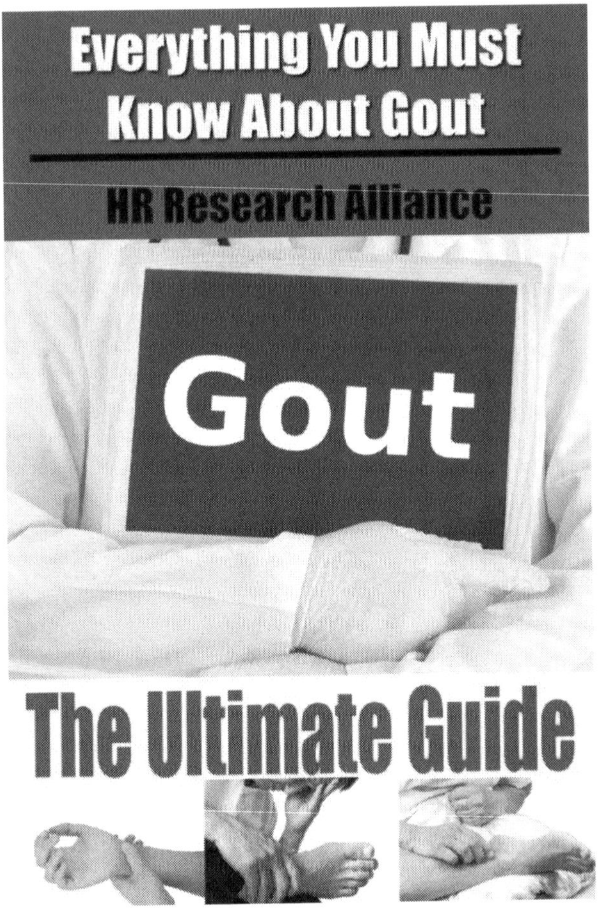
Everything You Must
Know About Gout
HR Research Alliance
Gout
The Ultimate Guide

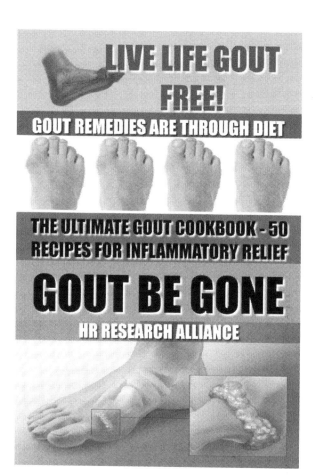

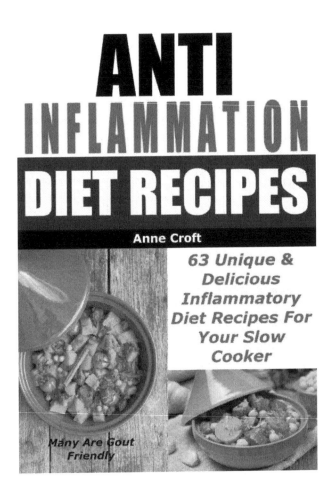

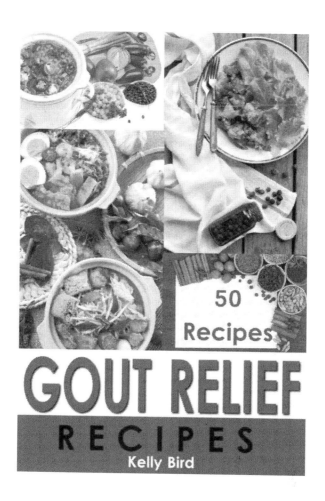

50 Recipes

GOUT RELIEF
RECIPES
Kelly Bird

This Book contains information that is intended to help the readers be better informed consumers of health care. It is presented as general advice on health care. Always consult your doctor for your individual needs. This book is not intended to be a substitute for the medical advice of a licensed physician. The reader should consult with their doctor in any matters relating to his/her health. No part of this Book may be reproduced or transmitted in any form or by any means, electronic or mechanical, including photocopying, recording or by any information storage and retrieval system, without written permission from the author.